UNDERSTANDING

LIP ENHANCEMENT PROCEDURES

FOR BEGINNERS

Unlock The Secrets To Achieving Fuller, Natural-Looking Lips With Expert Insights On Cosmetic Treatments, Safety, And Personalized Care

DR. ALICIA SONYA

CONTENTS

DISCLAIMER

The information provided in this book is for educational and informational purposes only and is not intended as medical advice, diagnosis, or treatment. Always consult with a qualified healthcare professional before beginning any therapy, practice, or lifestyle change.

The author and publisher of this book make no representations or warranties regarding the accuracy, applicability, or completeness of the content presented. While every effort has been made to ensure the information provided is accurate and up-to-date, the field of health and wellness is constantly evolving, and the reader is advised to use discretion and seek professional guidance as needed.

This book contains references to individuals, products, websites, organizations, or other entities solely for informational purposes. The author and publisher do not endorse, sponsor, or affiliate with any of these references, nor do they receive any benefit from their inclusion. The mention of any names, trademarks, or products does not imply any association or endorsement.

The use of this book is solely at the reader's discretion. Neither the author nor the publisher shall be held liable for any damages, loss, or injury resulting from the use or misuse of the information contained herein.

ABOUT THIS BOOK

Understanding lip enhancement procedures For Beginners "serves as an invaluable resource for anyone considering or practicing lip enhancement, addressing each aspect of these transformative procedures with depth and clarity. As lip enhancement continues to grow in popularity, this guide covers the ins and outs of these treatments, providing readers with comprehensive knowledge of their options, outcomes, and key trends in the industry.

This guide demystifies popular techniques, revealing how modern advancements focus on achieving natural-looking results and debunking common myths about enhancement procedures.

This book emphasizes informed decision-making, equipping readers with the knowledge they need to pursue their ideal results confidently.

A strong foundation in understanding lip anatomy is vital, and this guide dedicates itself to explaining the intricate structures that contribute to lip shape and appearance. By delving into the natural variations in lip shapes and how these structural differences influence enhancement possibilities, readers gain insight into how anatomy directly impacts the selection and success of treatments. An appreciation of individual features not only helps readers make informed choices but also highlights the significance of proportion and symmetry, essential components for achieving balanced and harmonious results.

This guide offers an in-depth look at the wide range of procedures available, from temporary fillers to permanent implants and fat transfers. Each option's benefits and potential drawbacks are analyzed, helping readers understand the different procedural outcomes and the importance of selecting the right method for their lifestyle and aesthetic goals. Recognizing that these decisions should be made in consultation with a professional, the book underscores the importance of expertise in enhancing both safety and satisfaction.

For those particularly interested in fillers, this guide offers a dedicated section exploring different filler types, injection techniques, and their unique advantages. Readers will discover what goes into creating results that look both natural and complementary, as well as what to expect in terms of maintenance, side effects, and recovery. This thorough approach provides transparency, allowing readers to prepare realistically for the experience and understand how proper aftercare contributes to a smooth healing process.

Beyond clinical procedures, this book explores non-invasive and at-home options that have become popular for their accessibility and lower cost. From lip-plumping serums to derma rollers, these methods are examined critically, noting how their results differ from professional treatments and their limitations.

This section enables readers to make well-informed choices about what works best for their needs, whether they seek subtle enhancement or simply want to experiment with at-home techniques.

Safety remains a primary concern in lip enhancement, and this guide dedicates significant focus to understanding the risks and potential complications involved.

By educating readers on the importance of choosing a qualified provider and recognizing the signs of possible complications, this guide serves as a reliable advocate for safety. Ethical considerations are also explored, reinforcing the necessity of professionalism and transparency within the industry.

Recognizing the diversity of individual needs and preferences, this guide includes a personalized approach to selecting enhancement techniques. It encourages readers to consider their aesthetic goals, age, lifestyle, and skin type in tandem with different procedural options.

By tailoring choices to individual features and realistic expectations, readers are empowered to achieve results that reflect their unique preferences and personalities. This section also prepares readers to communicate effectively with their providers, fostering collaborative discussions that lead to satisfying results.

In addressing common concerns and debunking persistent myths, this guide alleviates fears surrounding lip enhancement.

Misconceptions around unnatural outcomes, pain, and exaggerated side effects are dispelled with facts, giving readers a balanced perspective on what to realistically expect. This guide acknowledges the social and personal reservations that can accompany enhancement decisions and offers thoughtful insights to help readers feel more at ease with their choices.

For first-time clients, this guide is an essential companion, answering key questions about the preparation, procedure, and aftercare involved in lip enhancement.

From how to prepare before an appointment to the frequency of maintenance sessions and options for reversing results, this book provides crucial information to help newcomers feel comfortable and informed about their experience. It differentiates between temporary and permanent options, guiding readers in choosing the best fit for their desired commitment level.

Lastly, aftercare and maintenance are essential for achieving and preserving optimal results, and the guide offers expert advice on caring for enhanced lips. From avoiding certain habits to promoting hydration and planning touch-up appointments, readers receive practical tips on how lifestyle choices impact their outcomes.

This section encourages healthy practices that support both the longevity and appearance of enhanced lips, ensuring that readers are fully equipped to enjoy the results of their lip enhancement journey.

CHAPTER ONE

Introduction To Lip Enhancement

Lip enhancement refers to a variety of cosmetic procedures designed to enhance the shape, fullness, and definition of the lips. These procedures are popular for their ability to improve facial symmetry and add volume to the lips, making them look plumper and more youthful.

Over the years, the demand for lip enhancement has grown significantly, driven by the pursuit of a fuller and aesthetically pleasing smile that harmonizes with the rest of the face. While initially popular mainly in cosmetic circles, lip enhancements have become mainstream, with many looking to achieve subtle, natural-looking results.

There are several options available for lip enhancement, from minimally invasive injectables like hyaluronic acid fillers to more permanent solutions such as lip implants. Non-surgical options have been especially popular, as they offer less downtime and can be customized for different aesthetic goals. Other techniques, such as lip lifts and fat grafting, provide a more permanent or semi-permanent approach to lip enhancement, catering to various needs and preferences in terms of longevity and desired outcomes.

The benefits of lip enhancement go beyond aesthetics; fuller lips can help rejuvenate one's appearance and provide greater facial balance. However, misconceptions about exaggerated or unnatural results can make some people hesitant. In reality, most modern lip enhancement methods prioritize subtlety, aiming to enhance the lips in a way that looks harmonious and natural. This guide aims to demystify these procedures and provide clear information on the types of lip enhancements available, including what to expect from each method.

Overview Of Lip Enhancement And Its Popularity

Lip enhancement is among the most requested aesthetic procedures, known for its ability to refresh facial features and boost confidence. Many people seek lip enhancement to address naturally thin lips or lips that have thinned over time. Others look to balance asymmetries or create a more defined lip line.

Whatever the reason, lip enhancement offers customizable options that cater to different facial structures and aesthetic preferences.

The popularity of lip enhancements has soared, in part due to the visibility of celebrities and influencers who openly share their experiences. Social media has played a significant role in this trend, helping to normalize cosmetic enhancements and encouraging people to explore subtle aesthetic improvements. Today, lip enhancement is considered a versatile tool in the broader field of facial aesthetics, used by people of all ages to achieve a more youthful or proportionate look.

Lip enhancement techniques have evolved to allow for a more natural outcome.

Treatments are now more advanced, with medical professionals using techniques that complement individual facial features, enhancing the lips without an overdone appearance. This tailored approach has made lip enhancements appealing to a wider demographic, as people seek results that highlight their natural beauty while maintaining a realistic look.

Types Of Lip Enhancement Techniques

Several lip enhancement techniques are available, each offering different levels of volume, shape, and longevity. The most popular non-surgical option is lip fillers, commonly made of hyaluronic acid, which is naturally occurring in the body. These fillers are injected directly into the lips, where they add volume and hydration, creating a fuller, softer look. Lip filler treatments are temporary, usually lasting 6–12 months, making them ideal for those new to lip enhancement or who want to explore different looks over time.

For those seeking a more permanent solution, lip implants are an option. Implants are small, soft silicone tubes inserted into the lips via tiny incisions, providing a long-lasting increase in volume. Another semi-permanent technique is fat grafting, where fat is harvested from another part of the body (such as the thighs or abdomen) and injected into the lips. This option provides a natural feel and is generally longer-lasting than fillers, though it requires a minor surgical procedure.

In addition to these techniques, lip lifts are also available for people who desire a more defined Cupid's bow or less distance between the nose and upper lip. A lip lift is a surgical procedure that removes a small amount of skin just below the nose, lifting the lip upward and creating a more pronounced pout. Each method has its own set of benefits and ideal candidates, and it's important to discuss goals with a qualified practitioner to determine the best approach.

Key Benefits And Common Misconceptions

Lip enhancement procedures offer a range of benefits, from a boost in confidence to a more balanced facial appearance. One of the primary benefits is achieving fuller, more youthful lips that enhance the overall look of the face. For some, lip enhancements help restore the volume lost with age, while others benefit from the added definition and symmetry that can be achieved. These procedures are also relatively quick, with minimal recovery time for non-surgical options.

Despite these benefits, common misconceptions can deter some people from pursuing lip enhancements. A prevalent misconception is that all lip enhancements look exaggerated or unnatural. In reality, techniques like subtle lip fillers are highly customizable, allowing for gradual enhancement and natural-looking results. The skill and experience of the practitioner also play a key role in ensuring the outcome aligns with the individual's natural features.

Another misconception is that lip enhancement procedures are painful and high-risk. However, with modern techniques and numbing options, most patients experience only mild discomfort during the process. The non-surgical options also carry minimal risks when performed by a licensed and experienced professional. Understanding the reality behind these misconceptions can make it easier for individuals to consider the procedures and enjoy the benefits.

Trends In Natural-Looking Lip Enhancements

Today's trend in lip enhancement leans towards a natural, understated look rather than dramatic transformations. Many people now prefer subtle changes that accentuate their natural lip shape, adding just enough volume for a soft, youthful appearance. This trend has led to techniques like the "lip flip," which uses small amounts of Botox to relax the upper lip and create a slight lift without adding extra volume, making it popular for those looking for very subtle results.

Another approach to achieving natural-looking enhancements involves layering fillers in multiple sessions, creating gradual changes rather than a one-time transformation. This technique, sometimes called "microdroplet" or "microinjection," allows practitioners to add small amounts of filler incrementally. By carefully building volume over time, patients achieve a look that doesn't appear artificially plumped, maintaining harmony with other facial features.

Personalization is key to natural-looking results, as practitioners carefully consider factors like lip shape, skin tone, and overall facial balance. Advances in fillers and injectables also contribute to this trend by allowing practitioners to work with products designed for specific outcomes. Whether opting for a tiny volume boost or more noticeable fullness, natural-looking enhancements can be customized for a balanced, flattering result.

What To Expect From This Guide

This guide to lip enhancement provides practical insights into the full range of options available, from temporary solutions to more permanent enhancements. By understanding each technique, readers will be better equipped to choose the approach that best fits their aesthetic goals and lifestyle. For beginners, the guide offers a straightforward explanation of how lip enhancement works, including important details about recovery and what results to expect over time.

As lip enhancement procedures vary in terms of complexity and longevity, this guide also includes valuable tips on preparing for treatments and managing post-procedure care. This includes details on how to minimize bruising and swelling, which are common after injectable treatments, as well as understanding the typical healing process for surgical options. Knowing what to expect in terms of downtime and aftercare can help ensure a smooth experience and optimal results.

Finally, this guide addresses the role of the practitioner, emphasizing the importance of choosing a skilled and experienced professional for safe, natural-looking results. Different enhancement techniques require specific expertise, and this guide offers insights on how to select a practitioner who can deliver results tailored to individual facial features.

Armed with this knowledge, readers will feel confident in making informed decisions about their lip enhancement journey.

CHAPTER TWO

Understanding Lip Anatomy

To achieve successful lip enhancement, a basic understanding of lip anatomy is essential. The lips consist of several key structures, including the vermilion border (the outer rim of the lips), the cupid's bow (the upper lip's center curve), and the philtrum (the two lines running from the upper lip to the nose). Each of these areas contributes to the overall shape and aesthetic of the lips, and enhancing any part can change the lips' appearance. Knowing these regions and how they interact allows professionals to make subtle adjustments to improve the shape and fullness of the lips.

The muscles surrounding the lips, such as the orbicularis oris, also play a vital role. This circular muscle controls lip movement and is crucial in maintaining structure and support. When enhancing lips, understanding how fillers will affect this muscle is necessary to avoid an overly plumped or unnatural look. An understanding of these foundational elements helps practitioners determines where to place fillers or make incisions for maximum effect.

Additionally, factors like skin texture, hydration, and lip vascularity impact the outcome of lip enhancement procedures. Proper knowledge of the blood supply, for example, is essential to prevent complications like bruising or hematoma.

Having a comprehensive understanding of these anatomical details guides practitioners in creating natural, balanced, and safe enhancements tailored to individual facial structures.

Basic Anatomy Of The Lips And Surrounding Area

The lips consist of three main parts: the vermilion border, which is the outline of the lips; the cupid's bow, which is the prominent curve on the upper lip; and the philtrum, the lines extending from the nose to the upper lip. The main muscle called the orbicularis oris, surrounds the lips and controls their movement. Blood supply is plentiful in the lips, making them highly sensitive and responsive to treatments. Knowing these anatomical details is key to achieving balanced results in lip enhancement, as certain areas are more prone to bruising or swelling if improperly treated.

Lip Shapes And Individual Variations

Lips come in many shapes and sizes, varying greatly from person to person. Some people have fuller lower lips, while others have a more pronounced upper lip. The natural curvature of the cupid's bow, lip thickness, and width all influence the overall appearance of the lips. These variations are essential to consider when planning enhancements, as they guide practitioners in preserving the natural look of the individual's lips while adding volume or contour. Understanding these features helps ensure a tailored, natural-looking result.

How Lip Structure Affects Enhancement Options

The unique structure of each person's lips affects how they respond to different enhancement techniques. For example, thinner lips may require a different filler technique than fuller lips to avoid an unnatural appearance. People with asymmetrical lips may need more precision to ensure even results. Knowing the specific structure of the lips allows for more effective treatment plans, reducing the likelihood of complications like unevenness or exaggerated results. This careful consideration of anatomy leads to results that are proportionate, balanced, and aesthetically pleasing.

Why Understanding Anatomy Improves Results

Knowing lip anatomy enhances precision in lip augmentation, ensuring that changes made will look balanced and natural. When injectors understand exactly where to place fillers, they can enhance specific parts of the lips without overfilling, maintaining the lips' natural movement and avoiding the dreaded "duck lips" effect. Such precision also allows injectors to focus on symmetrical enhancements, working with each person's unique anatomy to improve aesthetic appeal.

Additionally, understanding anatomy allows professionals to anticipate how lip movement and daily expressions will influence the final result. When filler is added strategically to support muscle function and movement, the enhanced lips look good in both relaxed and dynamic states. By using their knowledge of underlying muscle patterns, injectors can balance aesthetic goals with natural expression.

Professionals with a solid grasp of anatomy also have better control over potential risks. They can avoid critical structures, ensuring that fillers are administered in areas with minimal vascular risk, reducing the chance of complications. A deeper understanding means that practitioners can confidently create results that align with both client desires and physiological needs, increasing overall satisfaction with the procedure.

Common Issues With Lip Symmetry And Proportion

One common issue in lip enhancement is maintaining symmetry, as many individuals naturally have slight asymmetries between the left and right sides of their lips. Injectors often adjust filler placement to balance these disparities, adding small amounts to one side to achieve a more harmonious look. Another factor is ensuring proportionality between the upper and lower lips, as lips with an exaggerated upper lip can look unnatural. Typically, the lower lip should be slightly fuller than the upper lip for the most natural appearance.

The shape of the cupid's bow is also crucial in creating visually appealing lips. Some people have a well-defined cupid's bow, while others have a flatter one, and this part can be adjusted during lip augmentation to suit the client's aesthetic preference. Maintaining a balance in the shape of the cupid's bow with the rest of the lips and face ensures a more natural, personalized look, with special focus given to preserving the individual's unique lip contours.

Finally, adjustments are often made to the lips' corners to ensure the lips have a slight upward tilt, creating a more youthful, relaxed expression. Overfilled or misaligned corners can lead to a "joker-like" appearance, so injectors need to be careful in this area. By understanding and addressing these common issues, practitioners can deliver well-proportioned, symmetric, and aesthetically pleasing lips that enhance the client's natural features.

CHAPTER THREE

Types Of Lip Enhancement Procedures

Lip enhancement procedures come in various forms, tailored to meet individual preferences and desired outcomes. Lip fillers, one of the most popular choices, involve injecting hyaluronic acid-based solutions into the lips to increase volume, shape, and symmetry. These filters are relatively quick and minimally invasive, offering immediate results with minimal downtime.

Another option is lip implants, a surgical approach involving the insertion of soft, silicone-based materials that create a permanent increase in lip volume. Fat transfer is another effective method, where fat from another part of the body is injected into the lips for a more natural and subtle enhancement.

Each procedure has unique characteristics and suits different goals. Lip fillers are best for those who want a quick enhancement with the option to dissolve it if the results are unsatisfactory. Implants, however, are ideal for those seeking a more permanent solution without frequent follow-ups.

Fat transfer is a longer-lasting option as well, but it uses the body's natural tissue, which appeals to those looking for an organic approach. The choice of procedure depends significantly on desired results, recovery time, and willingness to undergo repeat treatments or surgical interventions.

When considering these procedures, it's important to understand the potential outcomes, recovery expectations, and costs associated with each. Some people prefer non-permanent options to allow for flexibility in appearance changes over time, while others are looking for a one-time, permanent enhancement. Deciding on the right procedure involves considering both aesthetic preferences and lifestyle, so knowing what each option entails will guide a more satisfying choice.

Overview Of Popular Procedures: Fillers, Implants, Fat Transfer

Lip fillers, implants, and fat transfers represent the most commonly sought-after lip enhancement techniques. Fillers, made primarily of hyaluronic acid, are injected just below the skin's surface and allow practitioners to shape and plump lips with precision, achieving both volume and symmetry. This minimally invasive procedure has a quick recovery time, with results visible almost instantly and lasting several months to over a year, depending on the filler type.

Lip implants provide a more lasting alternative and involve inserting silicone-based implants via small incisions made in the lips. Though it requires surgical intervention, implants are resilient and don't require periodic touch-ups, offering a permanent solution for fuller lips. Fat transfer, or lipofilling, involves removing fat from an area like the abdomen or thighs and injecting it into the lips. This method combines a natural appearance with longer-lasting results, although it typically requires a more extended recovery period than fillers.

Each of these options varies in terms of longevity, costs, and recovery. Fillers are generally preferred for those testing out lip enhancement, while implants and fat transfers cater to people seeking a more permanent solution. Consulting with a qualified specialist can help you choose the best procedure to meet your unique needs, lifestyle, and budget.

Temporary Vs. Permanent Options

Temporary lip enhancements, such as hyaluronic acid fillers, allow individuals to experiment with fuller lips without committing to a permanent change. These fillers naturally dissolve within six months to a year, offering flexibility for those who may want to adjust their appearance over time. Temporary options also provide a lower-risk introduction to lip enhancement, as the procedure is quick, involves minimal downtime, and any unwanted effects can be adjusted or reversed by the practitioner.

Permanent solutions include options like lip implants and, to a lesser extent, fat transfer. Lip implants require a minor surgical procedure but deliver enduring volume and shape without the need for frequent touch-ups. Fat transfer, while technically a longer-lasting method rather than truly permanent, also provides a stable enhancement option, as the transferred fat integrates with the body's tissues. Permanent enhancements appeal to those looking for a long-term solution and are willing to undergo surgery for lasting results.

Choosing between temporary and permanent solutions depends on your comfort level, lifestyle, and aesthetic goals. Temporary fillers suit people wanting low-commitment enhancements with a more gradual, adaptable approach, while permanent options are better for those with a clear idea of their ideal look. Both options have their pros and cons, making a professional consultation valuable in finding the best approach for individual needs.

Pros And Cons Of Each Procedure

Each lip enhancement procedure comes with distinct advantages and disadvantages. Fillers offer versatility, with easily adjustable results, minimal downtime, and the flexibility to add volume as needed. However, fillers require maintenance every few months, which can become costly over time. Implants, on the other hand, offer a permanent enhancement without recurring treatments, but the surgery involves a longer recovery and may carry higher upfront costs and risks associated with any surgical procedure.

Fat transfer combines some of the benefits of fillers and implants by using the body's natural fat for a more organic and lasting result. Since it uses the body's tissue, fat transfer is well-tolerated, but the results can be slightly less predictable as some fat may be reabsorbed over time. Additionally, it involves a more complex procedure than fillers, as fat must first be harvested from another part of the body, extending both treatment and recovery time.

Deciding on the best procedure involves weighing the need for longevity, cost considerations, and personal tolerance for surgical procedures. Fillers may be ideal for those seeking low-commitment options, while implants suit individuals with a preference for enduring results. Understanding each procedure's trade-offs allows for a more personalized approach to achieving the desired lip appearance.

Key Factors To Consider When Choosing A Procedure

Several factors play an essential role in choosing a lip enhancement procedure, such as desired results, budget, and long-term commitment. If the goal is temporary enhancement with the option to adjust over time, fillers are generally the best choice. For those looking for a long-term solution and willing to undergo a surgical procedure, implants offer a stable and consistent option. Cost is also a consideration; fillers require periodic maintenance, while implants and fat transfers involve higher upfront costs but eliminate frequent re-treatment expenses.

Recovery time varies across procedures, which can impact your choice depending on lifestyle and commitments. Fillers allow for a quick return to daily activities, with minimal downtime, while implants and fat transfers may require several days to weeks for full recovery.

Individuals should also assess their comfort level with surgery, as implants and fat transfers require more significant interventions compared to fillers.

Considering potential side effects and recovery time can also guide your choice, as some procedures carry more risks than others. Consulting with a board-certified professional will help clarify these aspects and ensure that the selected procedure aligns well with individual needs, expectations, and lifestyle factors.

Importance Of Consulting A Professional
Seeking the guidance of a qualified, board-certified professional is critical before undergoing any lip enhancement procedure.

A professional will assess your facial structure, skin type, and aesthetic preferences, helping to recommend the most suitable option. Additionally, they can provide insight into expected outcomes, risks, and recovery times for each procedure, helping to set realistic expectations and avoid potential dissatisfaction.

An experienced practitioner ensures the procedure is performed safely, with a meticulous technique that minimizes the chance of complications. They will also offer valuable information on the type and quality of materials used, whether it's the right filler or implant type for your needs, ensuring long-lasting and satisfactory results. Professionals can discuss different types of anesthesia and pain management options as well, making the experience more comfortable.

Consulting with a specialist also opens up the possibility for a customized approach to lip enhancement, taking into account individual needs and aesthetic goals. This personalized guidance is invaluable, as it allows for an informed decision based on both practical considerations and a clear understanding of each procedure's nuances.

CHAPTER FOUR

Lip Fillers – A Detailed Look

Lip fillers are non-surgical cosmetic procedures involving the injection of hyaluronic acid or other filler substances to enhance lip volume, shape, and symmetry. Hyaluronic acid-based fillers are popular due to their ability to retain moisture, creating a fuller appearance while looking and feeling natural.

The filler is carefully injected into the upper and/or lower lips, allowing for targeted enhancement based on the client's aesthetic goals. This approach has become popular as it offers temporary, customizable results that can be adjusted over time according to preference and facial changes.

The procedure itself is relatively simple. The professional numbs the lip area using a topical anesthetic to minimize discomfort, then uses fine needles or cannulas (thin tubes) to inject the filler substance. The injector often uses a microdroplet technique, injecting small amounts to achieve gradual enhancement. This allows for a more natural look rather than an overly plumped appearance. During the procedure, the client can usually monitor the results with a mirror to make minor adjustments as needed, which helps to achieve the ideal lip shape and volume.

Results from lip filler injections last anywhere from six months to a year, depending on the product used and individual metabolism.

Fillers gradually dissolve over time, so maintenance treatments are necessary to keep the desired volume. Following the initial treatment, clients may need touch-ups every few months to maintain their appearance. Regular maintenance also helps avoid abrupt changes in lip fullness, enhancing the look more natural over time.

Different Types Of Fillers And Their Benefits

There are several types of fillers available, with hyaluronic acid-based fillers like Juvederm and Restylane being the most common due to their versatility and natural-looking results. These fillers are FDA-approved, provide immediate volume, and are known for their flexibility, allowing injectors to shape the lips precisely.

Collagen-based fillers, although less common now, are another option, but they have been mostly replaced by hyaluronic acid fillers due to improved safety and lower risk of allergic reactions.

Polylactic acid fillers, like Sculptra, offer a unique benefit by stimulating collagen production rather than merely filling the area, which can provide a more long-lasting effect. These fillers are used more for volume loss associated with aging rather than pure lip augmentation, as the results develop gradually. For those looking for a firmer look with long-lasting results, calcium hydroxylapatite fillers like Radiesse may be recommended, though they are typically used in other facial areas due to their dense texture.

The choice of filler depends on the desired effect, budget, and the injector's expertise. Hyaluronic acid fillers remain popular due to their reversibility—if the client is dissatisfied, an enzyme called hyaluronidase can dissolve the filler quickly. Each filler type has unique benefits, and discussing these with a trained professional helps tailor the procedure to individual goals and ensures the best possible results.

Injection Techniques For Natural Results

To achieve natural-looking lip enhancement, injectors often use a variety of techniques, choosing based on the client's anatomy and aesthetic goals. The linear threading technique is one of the most common; it involves injecting filler in a straight line along the lip border or within the lip body to create even volume and define the lip outline. Another popular technique is the "microdroplet" method, which injects very small amounts of filler to gradually enhance volume without creating a "duck-lip" appearance.

The "tenting" technique, or Russian lip technique, involves injecting vertically along the lip lines to create a plumper, heart-shaped look, emphasizing the lip peaks and giving the illusion of height. This is often chosen by clients who want a voluminous yet structured look. For those looking to enhance lip symmetry subtly, the "pillow" technique might be recommended, where small amounts of filler are injected into specific areas of the lips that need balancing without affecting the natural shape.

Combining these techniques can often yield the best results, as it allows for custom shaping and avoids overfilling one area. Skilled injectors will assess the client's facial proportions, natural lip shape, and overall aesthetic goals before choosing the techniques to be used, ensuring a harmonious and natural outcome.

Duration And Maintenance Of Filler Results

Lip filler results generally last between six to twelve months, depending on factors such as filler type, individual metabolism, and lifestyle. Hyaluronic acid fillers, which are temporary, tend to break down gradually, allowing for a soft return to natural lip volume over time. Those looking to maintain their enhanced lips often schedule maintenance treatments every six to nine months, though this varies depending on personal preference and desired fullness.

For those who want longer-lasting results, alternatives like semi-permanent fillers can be considered, but these often come with additional risks. Maintenance sessions are typically quicker and require less product than the initial treatment, making them convenient for clients who want consistent results with minimal interruption. During each session, injectors may make minor adjustments to refine the shape and balance, which helps in maintaining a natural appearance.

Proper aftercare and lifestyle can also impact the longevity of filler results. Avoiding extreme heat exposure, such as sunbathing or in hot tubs, and staying hydrated can help preserve filler effects. Consistent maintenance and appropriate aftercare support the longevity of fillers and contribute to the client's satisfaction with their enhanced appearance.

Possible Side Effects And Risks

While generally safe, lip fillers come with potential side effects and risks, including swelling, bruising, and tenderness at the injection site. Most of these side effects are mild and resolve within a few days. Some clients might experience temporary lumps or unevenness, which typically smooth out within a week. Rare but more serious side effects can include infection, vascular complications, or allergic reactions, though these are minimized when treatments are performed by licensed and experienced professionals.

In some cases, clients may experience what is called "vascular occlusion," where filler accidentally blocks a blood vessel, potentially leading to skin damage if not treated promptly. Injectors are trained to recognize early signs of this and have protocols to dissolve the filler if necessary, which is why seeking a certified professional is crucial.

An allergic reaction to the filler is rare, especially with hyaluronic acid-based fillers, but allergy testing can be done for additional safety if needed.

Clients should also be cautious about the potential for migration, where filler moves from the injection site to adjacent areas, leading to unwanted swelling or changes in shape. Keeping the lips hydrated, following aftercare instructions, and avoiding pressure on the lips in the days following treatment can help reduce these risks. Discussing potential risks and realistic expectations with a professional before treatment is essential for a safe and satisfying experience.

Recovery Process And Aftercare Tips

Post-procedure, some swelling, bruising, and tenderness are normal, and it may take up to a week for lips to settle fully. Applying ice packs to the lips intermittently can help reduce swelling and alleviate discomfort, but avoid putting too much pressure on the area. It's also recommended to sleep with the head elevated on the first night to minimize fluid accumulation and reduce swelling.

For the first 24 to 48 hours, it's best to avoid activities that increase blood flow to the face, like strenuous exercise, saunas, or hot baths, as these can exacerbate swelling and bruising. Staying hydrated, moisturizing the lips, and avoiding certain skincare products (like retinoids or AHAs) around the mouth are essential in supporting healing. Eating gentle, non-irritating foods can help avoid excessive lip movement, minimizing discomfort during the healing process.

Follow-up appointments allow the injector to assess healing and make any necessary adjustments. After the initial recovery phase, clients can resume regular lip care and enjoy their enhanced appearance. Following these tips not only ensures comfort but also enhances filler longevity, making the most of the investment in lip enhancement.

CHAPTER FIVE

Non-Invasive And At-Home Options

Non-invasive lip enhancement options have grown popular due to their convenience, affordability, and minimal risk compared to professional procedures. These methods often include the use of serums, natural techniques, and devices that can be incorporated into a daily routine. Unlike surgical procedures, non-invasive options do not provide permanent results but are ideal for those looking for a quick, temporary enhancement without any significant downtime or cost. They're best suited for those who want a natural, subtle boost without a dramatic change.

Among these options, lip-plumping serums and creams are commonly used as they are easy to apply and offer quick, albeit temporary, results. These products contain active ingredients like hyaluronic acid, menthol, or ginger that mildly irritate the lips, causing them to swell slightly, giving a fuller appearance. For application, it's recommended to start with clean lips, apply a small amount evenly, and wait a few minutes to observe the plumping effect. Most serums and creams provide effects that last for a few hours, making them a good choice for special events or daily use.

Additionally, there are at-home tools like derma rollers and suction devices. Dermarollers create tiny punctures in the lips to stimulate collagen production over time, which can lead to fuller-looking lips after consistent use. Suction devices work by temporarily drawing blood to the lips, creating a plump appearance, but they should be used with caution to avoid bruising. Both methods provide a temporary enhancement but should be used according to the manufacturer's instructions to prevent damage to the lips.

Lip-Plumping Serums And Creams

Lip-plumping serums and creams are popular for their simplicity and instant effects. They're easy to apply and generally made with ingredients that stimulate circulation or cause mild irritation, such as capsicum, menthol, or cinnamon oil, resulting in a fuller appearance. These products are widely available in most beauty stores, offering a variety of formulas and intensity levels, so beginners can find one that suits their preferences.

To use these products effectively, start by applying a small amount to clean, dry lips. Some products may provide a tingling sensation—this is a common effect of plumping agents, but it should be mild. Within minutes, you'll likely notice your lips appear fuller and more hydrated. However, because the plumping effect is temporary, you may need to reapply as needed for longer-lasting fullness throughout the day.

While effective for short-term results, these serums and creams do have limitations. Since their effects last only a few hours, they're best suited for temporary enhancement rather than long-term fullness.

Prolonged or excessive use can sometimes lead to lip dryness or sensitivity, so balancing use with moisturizing products is essential to maintain lip health.

Natural Techniques To Enhance Lip Volume

Natural methods to enhance lip volume are a practical choice for those looking to avoid artificial ingredients or tools. These techniques include massages, exercises, and using natural oils to improve circulation and hydration, creating the appearance of fuller lips over time.

Natural options offer a way to enhance lip volume gradually without relying on products or devices, making them ideal for those who prefer a gentle approach.

One effective technique involves using a soft toothbrush or a damp cloth to gently massage the lips in circular motions. This gentle exfoliation increases blood flow to the area, creating a temporary plumping effect. Additionally, regular lip exercises like puckering and holding or blowing kisses can help stimulate lip muscles, creating subtle fullness with consistent practice.

Using natural oils like coconut, almond, or peppermint oil can also add a hydrated and voluminous look to the lips. Peppermint oil, in particular, has mild tingling properties that can create a slight swelling effect. Applying these oils before bed and letting them absorb overnight can help maintain lip moisture and smoothness, giving lips a healthy, fuller look over time.

Tools And Devices: Dermarollers, Suction Tools

For those looking to take at-home enhancement step further, devices like derma rollers and suction tools can offer a more noticeable, though temporary, volume boost. Dermarollers work by creating tiny punctures in the skin, stimulating collagen production, and gradually leading to plumper lips with consistent use. Meanwhile, suction tools rely on vacuum-like pressure to increase blood flow instantly for a fuller appearance.

To use a derma roller safely on the lips, it's essential to start with a sanitized roller and clean lips.

Gently roll it over the lips in different directions, applying very light pressure to avoid injury. Afterward, applying a hydrating serum can help soothe the area and support collagen production. When used correctly, derma rolling can enhance lip volume subtly over time, but it should be done with care to avoid irritation.

Suction devices, while providing an immediate effect, are best used sparingly as overuse can cause bruising or damage to lip tissue. Begin by applying the device to clean, dry lips, and only use it for a few seconds at a time to avoid excessive suction. This method works best for temporary enhancement before a social event, but it should not replace more durable solutions for those seeking long-term fullness.

Comparisons To Professional Results

Non-invasive and at-home lip enhancement methods can provide some noticeable improvements but generally don't match the precision and durability of professional treatments like dermal fillers.

Professional lip fillers use hyaluronic acid-based injectables administered by trained practitioners, offering customizable results that can last for several months. In contrast, at-home methods tend to provide subtle, short-lived results that require frequent maintenance.

For those new to lip enhancement, at-home methods can serve as an introduction to achieving fuller lips without committing to a professional procedure.

These methods allow individuals to explore different levels of volume enhancement to decide whether they might want more significant changes later on. They're also typically more affordable, making them accessible to a broader audience interested in trying lip plumping on a budget.

However, it's important to note that at-home methods do have limitations in terms of safety and efficacy. Unlike professional treatments, they lack precision and often require multiple applications or careful handling to avoid potential side effects. Those seeking dramatic changes or long-lasting results may find professional treatments a more suitable and reliable choice in the long run.

Limitations Of At-Home And Non-Invasive Options

While non-invasive lip enhancement options are accessible and convenient, they come with limitations. The most notable drawback is the temporary nature of the results, which often last only a few hours. This means users need to reapply products or repeat treatments regularly to maintain the desired look, making these options better suited for short-term enhancement rather than a permanent solution.

Another limitation is the potential for side effects with frequent use of certain products or devices. For instance, continuous application of lip-plumping serums can cause dryness, sensitivity, or irritation, while improper use of suction tools might lead to bruising or skin damage. This makes it essential for users to carefully follow instructions and balance usage with nourishing lip care practices to avoid adverse effects.

Lastly, non-invasive methods lack the precision of professional procedures. At-home techniques cannot offer the tailored approach and control that a trained practitioner can achieve with injectable fillers. This means that those seeking a specific shape, symmetry, or lasting volume enhancement may find that professional treatments better meet their needs.

CHAPTER SIX

Safety And Risks Of Lip Enhancements

Understanding Potential Risks And Complications

Lip enhancement procedures, whether through fillers or implants, carry certain risks. The most common side effects include swelling, bruising, redness, and tenderness around the injection site.

In rare cases, more serious complications like infections, allergic reactions, or vascular occlusion (blockage of a blood vessel) may occur. These risks increase if the procedure is done incorrectly or by an untrained provider.

Importance Of Choosing A Qualified Provider

Choosing a certified, experienced medical professional is essential to minimize risks. Dermatologists, plastic surgeons, or licensed aestheticians with advanced training in injectables can ensure precise injections and reduce complications. They use quality products and adhere to hygiene standards. It's recommended to check the credentials, reviews, and before-and-after photos of your chosen practitioner to feel confident in your decision.

How To Reduce The Risk Of Side Effects

To prevent unwanted side effects, avoid alcohol, blood thinners, or anti-inflammatory drugs at least 24-48 hours before the procedure, as these can increase bruising.

Proper post-treatment care is also critical: applying ice, avoiding strenuous activities, and sleeping with your head elevated can help reduce swelling. If you notice severe pain, prolonged swelling, or unusual discoloration, seek medical attention immediately.

Signs Of Complications And When To Seek Help

Spotting Early Signs Of Complications
While some discomfort is normal, extreme swelling, excessive bruising, or hard lumps under the skin could indicate complications. Another serious concern is vascular occlusion, which can cause severe pain or discoloration if blood flow to certain areas is blocked. Infections may present with redness, warmth, and pus at the injection site.

When To Contact A Professional

It is essential to monitor your lips closely in the days following the procedure. If you experience symptoms like difficulty breathing, severe allergic reactions (anaphylaxis), or worsening pain, you should contact your provider or seek emergency medical care. Quick intervention can prevent permanent tissue damage or more serious health issues.

Follow-Up Care Matters

Make sure to attend follow-up appointments with your provider to ensure that healing is progressing smoothly. If adjustments are needed, such as dissolving excessive filler with hyaluronidase, this can be discussed during follow-ups. A good provider will ensure your satisfaction while prioritizing your health and safety.

Legal And Ethical Considerations

Regulations Around Lip Enhancement Procedures

Lip enhancements must follow strict medical regulations to ensure safety. In most countries, only licensed medical professionals can administer dermal fillers or perform lip surgeries. It is illegal to obtain or inject fillers from unverified sources or use non-FDA-approved products, as these may lead to severe complications.

Ethical Practices In The Industry

Ethical providers will conduct thorough consultations, discuss risks and realistic outcomes, and provide honest recommendations. They avoid pressuring patients into unnecessary treatments and will refuse procedures if they believe they compromise the patient's safety. A good provider will prioritize long-term health and natural results over short-term trends.

Patient Responsibility And Informed Consent

Before undergoing any lip enhancement, you'll need to sign an informed consent form. This document outlines the risks, benefits, and expectations of the procedure. Always read it carefully and ask questions if anything is unclear. Being fully informed helps you make the best decision while protecting your rights as a patient.

CHAPTER SEVEN

Personalized Lip Enhancement Choices

Selecting a lip enhancement procedure is highly individualized, beginning with understanding your specific preferences and goals. Each option, from temporary fillers to more permanent procedures, offers unique results tailored to different aesthetic desires. Some may want subtle volume, while others prefer a more defined shape or enhanced symmetry.

Start by identifying whether you're aiming for a plumper look, more definition, or simply a hydrated appearance—these preferences guide which procedure will work best.

Common procedures include injectable dermal fillers like hyaluronic acid, which add volume and definition, and more permanent options, such as lip implants, which provide a consistent plumpness over time.

Hyaluronic acid-based fillers are popular for beginners, as they're customizable and can be dissolved if desired. Each option varies in downtime and results in longevity, so understanding these factors is crucial to making a confident choice.

A thorough consultation with a licensed professional can help further refine your options. Providers will assess your facial structure, skin type, and enhancement goals, allowing them to recommend the best fit.

This process also includes determining the appropriate amount of filler or enhancement type, balancing your desired look with what will look natural and feel comfortable for your unique features.

How To Identify Your Goals For Enhancement

Identifying your lip enhancement goals is essential for achieving results that align with your aesthetic. Start by analyzing the current shape and size of your lips and decide if you want subtle adjustments or a more dramatic change.

Considering details like volume, contour, and symmetry can help clarify your vision and communicate it effectively to your provider.

Think about factors such as whether you prefer a noticeable or subtle enhancement, and consider how this might look in different lighting or angles. Collect photos of lip shapes you like, as well as those you don't, to provide clear visual references. Knowing what you want beforehand can help streamline the consultation process and ensure your chosen provider understands your expectations.

Once your goals are set, share them with your provider. They may recommend options that align with your vision or suggest alternatives based on your natural lip shape. An open discussion about your desired outcome and the steps involved helps manage expectations and ensures that you're on the same page before the procedure.

Matching Procedure Options To Personal Aesthetics

Matching your lip enhancement choice to your unique aesthetic ensures that the results will complement your overall appearance.

People with thin lips may benefit from subtle volume to achieve natural fullness, while those with asymmetrical lips might focus on balancing their shape. These preferences will often dictate whether temporary fillers, long-lasting injections, or even surgical procedures are the best fit.

Temporary fillers are ideal for those who desire versatility and the ability to modify or enhance their look over time. For a more permanent solution, procedures like fat transfer or lip implants can provide lasting results that suit those looking for a low-maintenance option. Matching the procedure to your aesthetic involves choosing techniques that suit your facial proportions, lifestyle, and willingness to maintain the results.

During your consultation, discuss how each option aligns with your lifestyle, as some procedures may require occasional touch-ups or maintenance. The right provider will help assess which approach best aligns with your aesthetic goals and overall lifestyle, ensuring that the outcome will look natural and blend seamlessly with your unique features.

Customizing Enhancement Based On Age, Skin Type, And Lifestyle

Customization in lip enhancement accounts for age, skin type, and lifestyle to create results that look natural and age gracefully. Younger individuals may seek mild enhancements for balanced proportions, while older clients often focus on restoring lost volume or addressing fine lines around the lips. Age impacts not only the choice of procedure but also the intensity of the enhancement required.

Different skin types react differently to fillers and implants. For example, those with sensitive skin may opt for gentler, temporary fillers that cause minimal irritation, while those with thicker skin may tolerate more robust procedures.

If you have an active lifestyle, consider how frequently you're willing to maintain enhancements, as some options require periodic touch-ups.

An experienced provider can guide the customization process, ensuring your enhancement aligns with both your aesthetic goals and practical lifestyle needs. They'll consider factors such as how a procedure may look over time, how your skin will respond, and what level of maintenance is feasible for you. This individualized approach creates results that look both flattering and natural at every stage.

How To Discuss Desired Results With A Provider

Communicating your desired results effectively with a provider is key to achieving your ideal lip enhancement.

Start by gathering reference images of the lip look you're aiming for, as these visuals can help avoid miscommunication.

During the consultation, discuss aspects such as volume, shape, and any particular preferences you have for symmetry or natural appearance.

Be clear about whether you want a subtle, natural enhancement or a more dramatic change. Your provider will likely guide you through what is achievable, explaining how your natural lip shape and facial structure affect the results. Understanding the different filler options, the effect of each, and the amount required for your desired look will also make this discussion more productive.

Being open about any concerns or reservations during the consultation allows your provider to address them in real-time.

They might suggest a gradual approach, starting with a smaller enhancement and adjusting over time. This conversation helps build trust and ensures that both you and the provider have aligned goals for the procedure.

Importance Of Realistic Expectations

Setting realistic expectations for lip enhancement is essential to avoid disappointment and ensure satisfaction with the results.

Recognize that enhancements will accentuate your natural features rather than completely alter them.

Most procedures, especially temporary fillers, provide subtle changes that blend with your appearance, enhancing your natural beauty without dramatic alteration.

Understanding that fillers and enhancements won't replicate another person's lips exactly helps manage expectations. Different procedures come with different levels of intensity, and some may require maintenance to preserve the desired look. Being open to a gradual enhancement can also provide a smoother transition to a new look that feels natural and comfortable.

Your provider will offer insight into what results can realistically be achieved based on your current lip shape, skin type, and age.

By establishing a clear understanding of what's possible, you're more likely to appreciate the result and avoid expectations that exceed what the procedure can deliver. Realistic goals ensure a positive experience and satisfaction with the enhancement over time.

CHAPTER EIGHT

Common Concerns And Myths

Addressing Fears Of "Fake" Or Unnatural Results

One of the most common concerns with lip enhancement procedures is the fear of unnatural or "fake" looking results. Many people worry that fillers will make their lips appear overly large or artificial. However, the outcome largely depends on choosing a qualified professional who understands facial aesthetics.

Skilled practitioners focus on symmetry and proportion, tailoring the amount and placement of filler to create a subtle enhancement that complements your unique features.

Additionally, modern lip fillers are designed to integrate smoothly with your natural lip tissue. By using hyaluronic acid-based fillers, which mimic substances already in your body, the results often feel and appear natural. It's also worth noting that the effect can be gradual; many practitioners offer a step-by-step approach, allowing you to add filler gradually over several sessions until you reach the desired look, minimizing the risk of an overdone appearance.

To prevent an unnatural look, have an open consultation with your practitioner about your goals. Bring reference images to clarify your ideal lip shape and fullness. Express concerns about overfilling, and be sure your provider respects your preference for subtlety.

Most experienced professionals aim for enhancements that leave clients looking refreshed, not altered.

Clarifying Myths Around Lip Fillers And Safety

There are widespread myths surrounding the safety of lip fillers, which can make people hesitant to try them. One common myth is that fillers are unsafe or "toxic." In reality, most fillers are made from hyaluronic acid, a naturally occurring substance in the body, making them safe for use.

When performed by licensed, experienced professionals, lip filler procedures are generally low-risk, and any adverse effects are usually minor and temporary.

Another myth is that once you start getting fillers, you must continue forever, or your lips will look worse. The truth is that fillers are gradually broken down by the body over time, so the results fade naturally without any negative impact on your natural lips. If you decide to stop getting fillers, your lips will simply return to their original shape without any sagging or thinning effects caused by the fillers themselves.

Finally, some people believe that all lip fillers are the same. Different types of fillers vary in thickness and durability, which can affect how the final results look and feel. Consulting with an expert who can recommend the best product for your needs ensures safer and more predictable results.

Concerns About Pain, Recovery Time, And Maintenance

Pain is often a top concern for those new to lip enhancement. Most fillers contain a numbing agent called lidocaine, and many practitioners apply a topical anesthetic before the procedure to minimize discomfort. While you may feel slight pressure or pinching, the process is generally quick, taking about 15-30 minutes. Pain is minimal for most people, and any lingering discomfort fades within a few hours post-treatment.

Recovery time for lip fillers is typically short, though some swelling and bruising can occur, lasting up to a week. Many people resume normal activities immediately after the procedure. To help reduce swelling, applying an ice pack and avoiding intense physical activity for the first 24 hours is recommended. Makeup can usually be applied the day after the procedure, allowing you to return to work or social events without obvious signs of enhancement.

Maintenance is straightforward, as most fillers last between 6-12 months. The longevity of your filler will depend on the type of product used, your metabolism, and your desired look. Touch-ups are typically needed once or twice a year to maintain fullness. Staying hydrated and avoiding smoking can also help prolong the life of your fillers, as these habits impact skin elasticity and filler breakdown.

CHAPTER NINE

Detailed Faqs For First-Time Clients

When considering lip enhancement, beginners often have many questions about the process. Lip enhancement, usually performed with injectable fillers, boosts lip volume, shape, and symmetry. For first-time clients, common questions include what to expect, pain level, duration of results, and the qualifications of the professional performing the procedure. It's also essential to understand the specific type of filler used, as some contain hyaluronic acid (HA), a natural substance that provides a fuller appearance while hydrating the lips.

In terms of safety, HA-based fillers are among the most common and widely tested for effectiveness and reversibility.

Procedures are generally minimally invasive, and while minor swelling or bruising may occur, they usually resolve within a few days. Clients can ask about numbing options, as some clinics offer topical anesthetics to make the procedure more comfortable.

To address specific concerns, clients should feel free to ask about costs, anticipated results, and post-care recommendations. Consulting with a licensed provider is crucial to address any allergies or skin conditions, and many providers offer a pre-treatment consultation to go over these details in person. Reliable practitioners will ensure clients feel informed and comfortable about every step.

How To Prepare For A Lip Enhancement Procedure

Preparing for a lip enhancement procedure begins with scheduling a consultation with a qualified professional who will assess your medical history, aesthetic goals, and expectations. It's essential to avoid certain medications, such as blood thinners or aspirin, for at least a week before the appointment to minimize the risk of bruising. Additionally, staying hydrated and avoiding alcohol or caffeine for at least 24 hours prior can reduce inflammation and enhance results.

On the day of your procedure, cleanse your face thoroughly, removing all makeup and skincare products around the lip area. Most practitioners recommend avoiding active skincare ingredients like retinoids for a few days before and after the treatment to prevent irritation. If you're prone to cold sores, let your provider know, as they may prescribe an antiviral medication to prevent flare-ups.

Finally, wearing comfortable clothing and arriving with time to relax will help calm any nerves. Some providers also encourage clients to eat beforehand since it's best to avoid applying pressure to the lips right after the treatment. A relaxed state allows the practitioner to assess your facial expressions and ensures you leave with balanced, natural-looking results.

What To Expect During And After The Procedure

During the procedure, a numbing cream is typically applied to the lips to minimize discomfort. Some dermal fillers also contain a mild anesthetic to ensure a more comfortable experience. The provider will use a fine needle or cannula to inject the filler strategically, focusing on specific areas to achieve the desired shape and volume. The process usually takes 15-30 minutes, and you'll be able to see initial results immediately.

Immediately after, you may experience some swelling, redness, or bruising around the injection sites. These side effects are normal and usually subside within a few days, although complete settling of the filler may take up to two weeks. During this period, it's recommended to avoid intense physical activity, excessive heat, and high-pressure areas, such as massages on the face, to prevent filler displacement.

For post-treatment care, you can use a cold compress to reduce swelling and avoid applying makeup directly to the lips for the first 24 hours. Most clients find any discomfort manageable with over-the-counter pain relief, and by following aftercare instructions closely, you'll ensure optimal results and minimal downtime.

How Often Do Results Need Maintenance?

Lip enhancement results generally last between six months to a year, depending on the type of filler used, individual metabolism, and lifestyle factors. Hyaluronic acid-based fillers tend to dissolve naturally over time, meaning regular touch-ups may be necessary to maintain the desired volume and shape. Lifestyle habits such as smoking, frequent sun exposure, and vigorous exercise can impact filler longevity, as they may accelerate the breakdown of HA in the lips.

Typically, practitioners recommend scheduling follow-up appointments every 6-12 months. Some clients opt for smaller, "maintenance" sessions at shorter intervals to keep their lips consistently full without major volume shifts. If the lips have completely returned to their natural state, a full enhancement session may be required.

When discussing maintenance with a provider, it's helpful to express any changes in aesthetic preference, as you may want to adjust the volume, shape, or specific areas targeted with each session. Consistency with a skilled professional ensures the most natural, balanced enhancements over time.

Can Lip Enhancements Be Reversed Or Adjusted?

Yes, most lip enhancements using hyaluronic acid fillers are reversible, which is beneficial for those new to the procedure or those who experience unexpected results.

If you're unhappy with the volume or shape, an enzyme called hyaluronidase can be injected to dissolve the filler within a few hours, effectively reversing the enhancement. This option is only available for HA-based fillers, as permanent fillers or implants are not reversible through the same method.

Adjustments, rather than full reversal, are often requested for refining or balancing results. In these cases, the practitioner may use a small amount of additional filler to perfect symmetry or shape. This is especially useful as natural facial asymmetry can sometimes be more noticeable after a filler procedure.

For clients considering reversibility, it's essential to choose a practitioner experienced in both filler application and reversal to ensure safety and satisfaction.

Always discuss these options during your consultation so you're fully aware of how to adjust your look if needed.

When To Choose Temporary Vs. Permanent Options

For beginners, temporary fillers are generally recommended, as they allow clients to experience lip enhancement without a long-term commitment. Temporary options, often hyaluronic acid-based fillers, provide subtle, natural-looking results that last between six months and a year. These fillers give clients the flexibility to change the look and adjust the volume as their aesthetic preferences evolve.

Permanent options, like lip implants, offer a solution for those who want a more lasting enhancement. However, these procedures are surgical, involve a longer recovery period, and may have more risks and complications.

Choosing permanent options is generally advised only for individuals who have experience with temporary fillers and are confident in their desired look.

In making this decision, it's vital to consult with an experienced provider who can discuss the pros and cons based on your facial structure, goals, and lifestyle. Many clients start with temporary fillers to achieve their ideal look before considering more permanent options, ensuring that the investment and results align with their preferences.

CHAPTER TEN

Aftercare And Maintenance For Lasting Results

Importance Of Proper Aftercare For Best Results

Proper aftercare is critical for ensuring the best outcomes after a lip enhancement procedure. Immediately following the treatment, you may experience some swelling or bruising, which is normal. Applying ice packs in intervals can help reduce swelling. It's also important to avoid touching or massaging the lips to prevent any unevenness in the filler. Keeping the area clean and avoiding makeup for the first 24 hours is essential for reducing the risk of infection.

Common Do's And Don'ts Post-Procedure

There are specific practices you should follow to ensure your lips heal properly. Do keep your head elevated while sleeping to reduce swelling. Avoid drinking alcohol and engaging in intense physical activity for at least 48 hours after the procedure, as these can exacerbate swelling. Don't expose your lips to excessive heat, such as saunas or hot showers, for the first few days. Refrain from smoking or using straws, as they can interfere with the healing process and the even distribution of the filler.

How Lifestyle Impacts The Longevity Of Results

Your lifestyle choices significantly affect how long your lip enhancement results last. Staying hydrated and maintaining a healthy diet rich in vitamins will help keep your skin and lips healthy. Avoid excessive sun exposure, as UV rays can break down the fillers faster. Regular skincare routines that involve moisturizing your lips will also help prolong the effects. Depending on the type of filler used, results may last anywhere from six months to a year, but maintaining a healthy lifestyle will help you get the most out of your procedure.

Tips For Keeping Lips Healthy And Hydrated

Daily Hydration Practices For Lips

Keeping your lips hydrated is key to maintaining their health and enhancing the appearance of your lip augmentation. Drink plenty of water throughout the day to keep your lips naturally moisturized from the inside out.

You can also use lip balms that contain hydrating ingredients like shea butter or hyaluronic acid to lock in moisture. Regularly exfoliating your lips gently with a soft toothbrush or a sugar scrub will remove dead skin cells, allowing lip balms to penetrate more effectively.

Avoiding Dryness And Irritation

To prevent dryness, avoid licking your lips, as this can remove natural oils and lead to chapping. Choose lip products that are free from harsh chemicals or fragrances that could irritate the sensitive skin on your lips.

If you're in a dry or cold climate, using a humidifier in your home can help add moisture to the air, reducing the risk of dry lips.

Sunscreen protection for your lips is also crucial, as UV rays can cause both dryness and accelerate the aging process.

Maintaining A Lip-Care Routine Post-Procedure

After a lip enhancement, it's important to incorporate new habits into your daily routine to maintain optimal results. Use a hydrating lip balm or treatment specifically designed to nourish and protect filler-enhanced lips. Avoid products containing menthol, eucalyptus, or other drying agents. Keep your lips moisturized, especially before bed, to avoid cracking. Eating a balanced diet and staying hydrated will keep your lips plump and healthy from the inside while using quality lip-care products will maintain the softness and appearance of your lips.

When And How To Schedule Touch-Up Appointments

Timing Your First Touch-Up

After your first lip enhancement procedure, your practitioner will likely recommend a touch-up within six to twelve months, depending on the type of filler used. It's important not to rush this process, as allowing the filler to settle over time will give you a clearer idea of how your lips respond to the procedure. During the touch-up, you can discuss whether you want to maintain your current volume or make slight adjustments.

Signs That A Touch-Up Is Needed

You'll know it's time to schedule a touch-up when you notice a gradual decrease in volume or fullness in your lips. Another sign is the reappearance of fine lines around the lips, which the filler was previously smoothing out. If your lips start to lose their symmetry or balance, a minor adjustment can help restore the desired shape. Keep in mind that scheduling regular touch-ups will keep your lips looking natural and refreshed without the need for a full procedure.

Coordinating With Your Practitioner

Always coordinate touch-up appointments with your original practitioner or a certified professional who has access to your treatment history. They will evaluate your lips and recommend whether more filler is necessary or if it's time for a break. The touch-up process usually involves less product than the initial procedure and takes less time. Be sure to plan your appointments at least a few weeks before any major events to allow healing time.

Conclusion

In conclusion, lip enhancement procedures have grown in popularity, offering a range of options to achieve fuller, more defined lips tailored to individual aesthetic goals. The variety of available techniques—from temporary solutions like dermal fillers to more permanent options such as lip implants—allows patients to select treatments aligned with their comfort level, budget, and desired longevity of results.

Minimally invasive treatments like hyaluronic acid-based fillers remain the most popular choice due to their relatively low risk, short recovery time, and reversibility, providing a suitable option for those new to cosmetic enhancements. For individuals looking for a long-lasting solution, procedures like fat grafting or lip implants can offer a more durable result, though they often involve more extensive planning and recovery.

Choosing the right procedure depends on several factors, including age, skin type, and overall health. Consulting a board-certified professional with experience in lip enhancement is essential to understanding the benefits and limitations of each technique and to ensuring a safe and satisfactory outcome. Thorough discussions with a professional help manage expectations and guide patients toward the method that best suits their needs and lifestyle.

It's also essential to consider potential risks, such as allergic reactions, asymmetry, and infection, although these are rare when performed by qualified practitioners. Additionally, post-procedure care is crucial for maximizing results and minimizing complications. Simple aftercare routines, such as avoiding certain activities or products, can significantly enhance the longevity and appearance of the enhancement.

Overall, lip enhancement offers transformative aesthetic possibilities. With the right preparation, realistic expectations, and a skilled professional, individuals can achieve beautiful, natural-looking results that enhance facial harmony and boost confidence.

Each procedure, from temporary fillers to permanent implants, has its unique advantages, making it possible to customize lip enhancement to any individual's personal beauty goals.

THE END